Table Of Contents

Abnormal Uterine Bleeding Treatment - Medication and Surgery

1. Introduction to Abnormal Uterine Bleeding

Abnormal uterine bleeding refers to changes in the pattern, frequency, and amount of menstrual flow and may be associated with excessive volume or duration of bleeding or both. AUB is a common gynecologic complaint that often significantly impacts the ability of premenopausal and perimenopausal women to function in their professional or personal lives. Lack of effective treatment for AUB, particularly in this group of women, may result in iron-deficiency anemia and poor quality of life. The treatment of AUB is patient-specific and includes medical, surgical, and device management. The extent to which each of these options is appropriate rests on the healthcare needs, wishes, and desires of the patient. Management is available with medications or surgeries, with the following common recommendations considering current medical practices, published resources from professional associations, and expert commentary.

Abnormal uterine bleeding (AUB) is a common gynecologic complaint that often significantly impacts the ability of premenopausal and perimenopausal women to function in their professional or personal lives. This topic page discusses medications used to help treat AUB when medication does not provide sufficient relief and the role of surgery to help these women lead normal lives.

2. Causes and Risk Factors of Abnormal Uterine Bleeding

The following are important points for evaluating a patient with abnormal uterine bleeding: The amount of blood lost during a normal menstrual period is 25 to 60 milliliters, or about 3 to 5 tablespoons. Many women complain their bleeding is excessive when the actual blood loss is normal. Subjective complaints may be most helpful in determining excessive blood loss. The frequency of tampon use is estimated by asking about the number of tampons or pads used. A patient using more than 20 or 30 tampons or pads a month may be donating blood to the local blood bank! Again, no absolute number defines an abnormal flow. The medical problems associated with abnormal uterine bleeding range from a benign process to endometrial cancer.

Doctors don't have a clear definition of what "normal" bleeding is for an individual. Many studies are done on the general public. However, it is likely that an individual knows when her bleeding is abnormal. She knows when her feminine protection products are soaked very quickly. She knows when she floods (soaks through her clothes and underwear). She knows when she is trapped at home or embarrassed about going out.

3. Diagnosis and Evaluation of Abnormal Uterine Bleeding

The specificity of a known cause for abnormal uterine bleeding determines the level of investigation that is appropriate. Primary care providers are generally capable of addressing most menstrual abnormalities. Family planning clinics and internal medicine healthcare providers also typically manage the evaluation of menstrual complaints. Urogynecologists and gynecologic oncologists specialize in the evaluation of abnormal uterine bleeding. Patients with a neoplastic, endocrinopathic, or refractory ovarian function problem will need to see an endocrinologist or a molecular geneticist. Patients at high risk for cervical cancer or gynecologic or endocrinologic malignancy will be referred to specialists for additional testing.

Menstrual patterns are often so individual and unique that it is hard to know what is normal and what is not. Some women do not keep track of their periods, and what can be a normal length for some may seem abnormal to others. Menorrhagia is heavy flow (e.g., requires a woman to change a pad or tampon every 1-2 hours) that can lead to anemia. Metrorrhagia is bleeding at irregular intervals, particularly between menstrual cycles. Menometrorrhagia is prolonged or excessive uterine bleeding. Tuberculosis, endometritis, adenomyosis, fibromyomas, and polyps, and PCOS are causes of irregular bleeding. Among the considerations of menstrual disorders is the necessity to rule out neoplastic, endocrinopathic, and other significant organic disease.

4. General Treatment Approaches

In summary, the treatment of AUB requires a comprehensive approach that takes into account the individual needs and circumstances of each woman. By considering the various treatment options available and involving women in the decision-making process, healthcare providers can work towards effectively managing AUB and improving the quality of life for women affected by this condition.

For most women, the primary treatment goal is to minimize the number of days with bleeding, particularly for those experiencing severe PB. It is important to achieve rapid symptom improvement while ensuring long-term effectiveness. Involving women in the decision-making process helps in implementing treatment plans and ensures that potential underlying pathologies are not overlooked. Understanding the natural progression of AUB in a woman and its underlying causes is crucial for selecting appropriate treatment options. Therefore, a four-level plan of action is generally followed in treatment: first, providing general advice on premenstrual awareness, fertility, abstinence, or contraception; second, if AUB recurs, prescribing a course of non-steroidal anti-inflammatory drugs that are tailored to the woman's life cycle and do not have genotoxic effects; third, if problems persist, ablative procedures with moderate effectiveness and objective measures of benefit but unknown long-term durability may be considered; and finally, if problems persist or recur after ablation, further treatment options should be defined.

Abnormal Uterine Bleeding (AUB), historically known as anovulatory metrorrhagia (AM) or dysfunctional uterine bleeding (DUB), refers to vaginal bleeding from the uterus that is irregular in terms of frequency, duration, or volume. There are different presentations of AUB, including heavy and prolonged bleeding periods (PB) or episodes of bleeding that occur more frequently and are separated by varying lengths of time (irregular intermenstrual uterine bleeding - IM). The underlying causes of AUB can vary, especially based on the woman's age. Currently, there is no single medical therapy or drug treatment that effectively addresses all aspects of AUB, which can have a significant impact on a woman's physical, emotional, social, and material well-being.

5. Medication Options for Abnormal Uterine Bleeding

3. The Levonorgestrel-Releasing Intrauterine System (IUD) - A small T-shaped device is placed in the uterus. It releases a small amount of progestin each day directly to the lining of the uterus, resulting in the length and amount of bleeding you have over time.

2. Progestin-Only Methods - These methods include pills, injections, implants (Nexplanon), and IUDs. Progestin-only methods can be used to reduce menstrual bleeding and may also help to relieve heavy cramping.

1. Combined Hormonal Birth Control - It contains two hormones - estrogen and progestin. It can help to regulate your menstrual cycle and reduce blood flow. It can also help to relieve the pain of menstrual cramping.

Many different medications can be used to help with abnormal uterine bleeding (AUB). Your doctor will use a combination of your symptoms, your age, your overall health, any future pregnancy plans, and any risks to treatment to help decide which medication is best for you. In this section, we will review many different medication options that are commonly used for AUB.

5.1. Nonsteroidal Anti-Inflammatory Drugs (NSAIDs)

The use of cyclooxygenase inhibitors in combination with select estrogens can be used to modulate vascular permeability, control uterine bleeding, and enhance potential anti-proliferative or pro-apoptotic response. Theoretically, early onset of cyclooxygenase inhibitor use might help prevent the establishment of irregular bleeding from anatomic or thrombotic events like HMB with secondary iron-deficiency anemia late in the menstrual life period. Their use during pregnancy might also reduce the risk of placental complications like growth deficits, abruption, and uteroplacentalopathy.

Although most NSAIDs have potent uterine stimulatory effects, they do not have the inherent abuse potential of a potential cancer chemopreventive agent like an aromatase inhibitor. NSAIDs are extremely effective for the immediate management of acute bleeding, premenstrual bleeding, or symptomatic bleeding from submucosal fibroids or endometrial polyps. The combination of a cyclooxygenase inhibitor for immediate relief of cramping, sudden onset, or moderate to severe bleeding, and continued pretreatment for a sustained reduction of blood loss, has been shown to be most effective. Hormonal or non-hormonal treatments can also be given in conjunction with a cyclooxygenase inhibitor to suppress monthly uterine bleeding by 50-90%. Since fibroids can grow and become more symptomatic with age, providing contraceptive and/or estrogen replacement benefits for women on long-term cyclooxygenase inhibitor therapy or cessation of use, they have decided to build families or achieve a menopausal state.

5.2. Oral Contraceptives

Periodic rather than daily use of such medication can provide regular cycles. Often these medications are given for 21 days, and it is the withdrawal of the hormone that induces the bleeding episode. They can provide predictable schedules and supportive care for 28-day cycles or comparable schedules. Administering such medications to adolescent females, the typical pattern of menstrual difficulties (cramping, excessive flow, and interval) does not change despite the fairly consistent non-contraceptive request. Just what the request is changes. If it truly reflects the patient's goals and acceptance of the potential complications of these medications, then by all means use them. Doses of hormone are not the same for women desiring only contraception vs women desiring menstrual cycle predictability. Penissticks or comparable dose hormones used in such doses are not always supplied in oral contraceptive containers or packs. However, physicians can prescribe the necessary doses by prescribing estrogen doses of 35 pg or seven ethinyl estradiol daily for 21 days, followed by five or other similar oral contraceptive.

Estrogens and progestins are used in oral contraceptives for contraception. When given to women not requiring contraception, oral contraceptives can reduce menstrual blood flow and provide predictable cycles. An advantage of their use in medications for abnormal uterine bleeding is that they do at least prevent endometrial cancer in patients with an intact uterus, preventing hyperplasia that might otherwise occur.

5.3. Progestin Therapy

Intrauterine The option of intrauterine progestin is also available. Levonorgestrel is the type usually provided. The IUD works by reducing bleeding, but it is not commonly used for long-term suppression. When the medical therapy fails, a patient might be counseled about the use of long-acting reversible contraception. However, the IUD is an option for patients who are interested in achieving amenorrhea and do not require long-term therapy. However, with either progestin or levonorgestrel, breakthrough bleeding can lead to amenorrhea. In those who still have pain, more aggressive evaluation must be made. With time, growth is needed, but this can cause endometrial progress. Before levonorgestrel treatment is started, polyps and hyperplasia must be absent.

Parenteral The progestin depot given intramuscularly is also an effective treatment. Medroxyprogesterone acetate is given as 150 mg every 3 months. Alternatively, a newer depot is used that is injected subcutaneously. This formulation consists of 104 mg of levonorgestrel and can be delivered with an autoinjector. Users need to have proper bone density and health, no undiagnosed uterine bleeding, and good cholesterol levels. A concern in these users over time is that body weight will begin to rise, which could negatively impact the metabolic syndrome. When bone density is questioned, it is crucial to track it. It is a decrease in response to a progestin effect, but when the progestin stops, the bone density may return.

Oral Options Progestin can be given orally in the form of medroxyprogesterone acetate at a dosage of 10 mg/day for 14 days, repeated every 1 month for a total of 3-6 cycles. Another option is norethindrone at a dosage of 2.5-5 mg/day for 7-10 days, repeated every 1 month for up to six cycles. Once therapy ends, amenorrhea or recurrent abnormal uterine bleeding may be noted. Another option is the use of continuous administration of norethindrone in a dosage of 1-2.5 mg/day for 20-40 days each month. Dinogest is a newer progestin that is used for longer-term suppression and is active by mouth at a dosage of 2 mg/day for an extended time period. A relatively new progestin called drospirenone has been developed for long-term treatment of PMB at a different dosage tab and cycle length as well.

Progestin therapy can be achieved through the use of oral, parenteral, and intrauterine routes. Systemic progestin therapy can reduce endometrial growth and limit abnormal bleeding, while an IUD containing levonorgestrel can suppress and atrophy the endometrium.

5.4. Tranexamic Acid

Two systematic reviews of the use of tranexamic acid for the treatment of heavy menstrual bleeding were published in 2006. Both reviews include the same two trials, but the more recent review incorporated additional evidence including the result of trials reported in abstracts. In two trials involving a total of 691 women, the effect of various doses of oral tranexamic acid was assessed. A possible effect on menstrual blood loss was suggested; compared with placebo, the red blood cell loss was reduced by 2.48 ml to 48.7 ml with the 2 to 4 gm/day dose, and 0 to 46.7 ml with the 1.5 to 3 gm/day dose. In one of the trials, some treatments were not reported, and data on both the quantity and duration of bleeding were not fully reported. Minor side effects were reported, but no major adverse events were attributed to the therapy.

Tranexamic acid is an antifibrinolytic that inhibits clot degradation. It is thought that patients with heavy menstrual bleeding have increased fibrinolytic activity that contributes to the excessive blood flow. Tranexamic acid reportedly has a positive effect on heavy menstrual bleeding. Two trials involving a total of 691 women with heavy menstrual bleeding showed that tranexamic acid reduced menstrual blood loss. On the basis of these findings, we believe that tranexamic acid is beneficial for women with heavy menstrual bleeding.

5.5. Gonadotropin-Releasing Hormone (GnRH) Agonists

Gonadotropin-releasing hormone agonists are medications that are similar to, but stronger than, gonadotropin-releasing hormone. It is not understood how these medications work in treating fibroids or endometriosis. Gonadotropin-releasing hormone agonists are sometimes given for 3 to 6 months before surgery to shrink the fibroids. They can also be used to keep a woman from having her period. This can improve the blood count and prevent blood transfusions in a woman with very heavy menstrual periods. Weight gain, decreased bone density, hot flashes, and depression are common side effects. If a woman uses this medication for longer than six months, she should take a small dose of estrogen. Taking a regular or high dose of estrogen can cause the fibroids to grow. As with many of the medications used to treat endometriosis, the symptoms may return after the medication is stopped.

5.5. Gonadotropin-Releasing Hormone (GnRH) agonists

5.6. Danazol

Danazol is no longer commercially available in the UK, but can still be obtained in Germany and other countries. It is not licensed for the treatment of AUB and is not routinely considered for use in the UK. However, individual clinicians may feel that danazol's utility as a non-contraceptive-contraceptive, if used judiciously, supports broader access within national healthcare systems. For example, women suffering from idiopathic AUB might ask for the temporary use of danazol if bleeding disturbed a vacation in which insertion of an IUS was physiologically inappropriate, because they do not wish to have systemic hormone therapy, or if they suffered from hormonal side effects. Similarly, danazol is often recommended for women who experience heavy or painful menstruation and in whom other medical options (eg NSAID or LNG-IUS) are not suitable, are contraindicated, or have failed.

Danazol is a synthetic steroid with some weakly androgenic and anabolic properties. The exact mechanism of its action is uncertain, but it may help to reduce dysfunctional uterine bleeding by improving the regulation of Gn. The majority of RCTs of danazol in idiopathic AUB have examined regimens comprising 20 to 600 mg danazol per day for ten to 28 days beginning either on day 16 of the cycle or when bleeding commenced. In these studies, danazol-containing schedules produced lighter, shorter, and less painful bleeding for up to three menstrual cycles, but the substances caused numerous side effects. Prolonged use is associated with weight gain, fluid retention, acne, hirsutism, muscle cramps, vaginitis, and a visible increase in skin sebum levels. Hormonal side effects reported from the use of danazol are hot flushes, sweating, excessive body hair growth, voice deepening, and clitoral growth; reversible elevation of HDL cholesterol and reversible therapy-related increase in triglycerides; and a reversible decrease in luteinising hormone and FSH levels and menstrual disturbances after the end of treatment, especially during the first ovulation cycle.

6. Surgical Treatment Options for Abnormal Uterine Bleeding

In addition to potential health problems, women's bleeding may sometimes have significant emotional, practical, and lifestyle issues that can profoundly impact the quality of women's lives. While many with AUB need surgery, several of them will benefit from medical therapy initially to control their symptoms, particularly if they are not at immediate risk for serious hematological complications. Overall, the treatment plan includes diagnosis and reassurance first, with any serious illnesses being ruled out and patients' concerns and desire for treatment being acknowledged and appreciated. Only then should the proper therapy be considered.

In women with AUB who have had surgery, represent a referral, have coexisting medical conditions that predispose to surgery, or are at high risk for bleeding or anemia, treatment with certain surgical management strategies is necessary. Often, the best therapeutic approaches.

In most women with AUB, particularly when a lesion is causing the bleeding, treatment with hormonal therapy, NSAIDs, or a levonorgestrel-releasing IUD (LNG-IUD; levonorgestrel = progestin) offers a reasonable opportunity for clearly defined improvement or resolution and obviates the need for surgical intervention. The choice of medical therapy depends on the cause of the bleeding, the underlying medical conditions, the woman's attempt to conceive, and the patient's personal preferences. As always, the status of contraception must be ascertained in women of reproductive age, and the options that are acceptable to the woman must be discussed. More advanced and expensive medical therapies are available and should be considered in those with failed first- or second-line therapy measures or in those women who have contraindications to first- or second-line therapies.

6.1. Dilation and Curettage (D&C)

There are several procedures that can be performed: hysteroscopy, dilation and curettage. The hysteroscopy is a thin flexible tube with a light and an optic that allows you to look into the uterine cavity and remove polyps, fibroids, small tactile biopsies (which allow the use of ultrasound guidance for other treatments). In the dilation and curettage, the cervix is dilated and the contents of the uterus are scraped out. This can be helpful in the premenopausal woman who has heavy bleeding. The success of helping the bleeding is dependent on whether an underlying disease process is helping provoke this heavy lesion that continues to cycle.

There are a number of ways one may surgically treat abnormal uterine bleeding. First, by understanding what the lining of the uterus is and how it relates to menstruation. The lining of the uterus is hormonally stimulated in preparation for a pregnancy. If pregnancy doesn't occur, this lining is shed. The menstrual period is the shedding of that lining. Treatment of the abnormal bleeding that occurs can be as simple as utilizing any one of the oral contraceptive pills. These are especially helpful if the patient is premenopausal and desires the ability to become pregnant. The other medications that can be helpful here are progesterone agents given in high doses, such as Medroxyprogesterone acetate (Provera). These medications can be helpful in pre-menopausal and postmenopausal women.

6.2. Endometrial Ablation

In properly selected patients, ablation may cure heavy dysfunctional uterine bleeding by treatment of the surface tissue within the uterus. This method of treatment is not the best approach for many pathologic bleeding uterine causes because of a lack of means of obtaining histopathological diagnosis with tissue creation. Such patients might have tissue embedded in the uterine muscle that is not contained within the endometrial cavity, and all potential anatomic or physiologic causes of menorrhagia are not identified by merely addressing the superficial innermost uterine lining tissue. Other commonly present uterine growths other than adhesions or scars can be at the cornual region where the tubal openings are causing severe bleeding and the possibility of hydrosalpinges or tuboovarian infections. If the intrauterine pressure of the fluid with tissue debris and clots is excreted into the more dilated fallopian tubes, a nag of infertility treatment and health concerns can be created. The adenomyotic, which describes endometrial tissue deep within the myometrium, may be a marker of a special entity that should be removed by a more definitive treatment.

This procedure is done under general anesthesia or local anesthesia with sedation. After the procedure is performed, patients should be advised that pregnancy may be possible because the uterine wall is preserved.

A very commonly performed office or outpatient surgery is performed for women with abnormal uterine bleeding arising from benign conditions of the uterine cavity. Global endometrial ablation is an outpatient surgical procedure that is performed by several methods, which include vaginally utilized thermal balloon containment of heated fluid, freezing temperature-induced destruction of the endometrium by uterine cavity administered liquid nitrogen or pipodium gel, rollerball or ball end diathermy electrical power application, microwave-induced destruction of cells, radiofrequency delivered cell destruction, laser spherical beam application, and mesh-contained thermal energy application. The aim of surgery is to destroy the endometrial tissue or the part of the uterine lining that makes monthly periods. Most patients will have either lighter or no menstruation after surgery but not a cure for their menorrhagia.

6.3. Hysterectomy

Hysterectomy performed for abnormal uterine bleeding is considered the definitive treatment. Women must be educated about the expected changes to menstrual flow/patterns associated with age as well as the methods and options available, and the risks/costs that can be expected with the menopause. They must have also discussed other options with their healthcare professional other than a hysterectomy option performed. The majority of hysterectomies being performed currently are the definitive solution meant for this problem. More than 600,000 hysterectomies are performed in the US for benign disease each year. Abnormal uterine bleeding, often initially treated conservatively with hormones or other office-based therapies, accounts for a large number of these hysterectomies. Between 2006 and 2011, 15% of the hospital admissions for abnormal uterine bleeding led to a hysterectomy. Between 2007 and 2013, the rates of hysterectomy performed for abnormal uterine bleeding did decrease by 3:1. However, a closer look demonstrated that the rate of change was only half of 1% per year. The decrease occurred entirely in white women ages 18-45, particularly advanced age of 40.

Hysterectomy performed for abnormal uterine bleeding includes removal of the uterus by open or minimally invasive method. The Fallopian tubes and ovaries can be conserved or removed based on the woman's clinical condition. Several alternative nonhysterectomy options are available and women must be fully supported to explore these options, unless there is no such possibility for a successful outcome, or an emergency like bleeding is happening. The gold standard surgical option remains total abdominal hysterectomy at this time, as it has been performed for years and there is more data on its safety, efficacy, and outcomes. Minimally invasive hysterectomy approaches, like using laparoscopy (total or subtotal) or robotic technology (total or subtotal), are available at some locations but are not as commonly done due to several reasons including lack of familiarity and skill at all hospitals and not every woman being a candidate for these approaches.

7. Minimally Invasive Procedures for Abnormal Uterine Bleeding

Endometrial ablation is most effective for those with heavy menses and regular periods; however, this is not a safe option for those with anatomic abnormalities. For example, adenomyosis, which is when endometrial tissue grows into the muscle layers of the uterus, or fibroids that encroach into the uterine cavity can mimic symptoms of heavy bleeding and generally are resistant to endometrial ablation. Most patients can resume normal activities within a day or two, although they may have some vaginal discharge for a few weeks. Some patients may experience mild cramping the day of the procedure. For 5 to 10 percent of the women who have the procedure, bleeding does not disappear and a second procedure or possibly a hysterectomy is necessary. In a young woman, heavy menstrual periods are common. Proper screening and testing is essential because endometrial ablation should only be done for people who have completed childbearing.

For select cases of persistent or recurrent abnormal uterine bleeding, an outpatient minimally invasive procedure to thin the lining of the uterus may be recommended. This procedure specifically targets the lining of the uterus and is an alternative to hysterectomy. The endometrial layer is treated and usually does not regrow. The most appropriate candidates for endometrial ablation are those who have heavy bleeding with regular menses because ablation cannot remove large fibroids. To perform endometrial ablation, the cervix is gradually dilated and the endometrial lining is visualized with a hysteroscope. A physician trained in minimally invasive procedures then applies various techniques to the endometrial lining, virtually eliminating it. The procedure takes only about 15 minutes and is performed in a doctor's office or in an outpatient center, depending on the technique used. No hospitalization is necessary and recovery is usually minimal.

7.1. Hysteroscopy

Hysteroscopy may be performed in different time settings: in the office, ambulatory surgery, or in an in-hospital scenario. Office-based hysteroscopy is performed using a small gauge hysteroscope and allows the performance of the technique in generating visual acuity comparable with the hospital-based approach. Consequently, office-based hysteroscopy is cost-effective and less morbid, requires no general anesthesia, and has the potential to replace hospital-based procedures in the future. Proper instrumentation and anesthetics are mandatory. However, in 2013, the Consensus en Histeroscopia en la Atención Primaria declared: "Office hysteroscopy should become a standard procedure for primary care clinics providing care for peri- and postmenopausal women treated especially with hormonal replacement therapy".

Hysteroscopy has become the standard tool for the diagnosis of intrauterine pathology, allowing resolution of a wide range of intrauterine disorders. Also, hysteroscopy is an interesting modality in the treatment of intrauterine abnormalities that previously were treated by laparotomy or laparoscopy with increased morbidity and costs. Overall, hysteroscopy has reduced morbidity, making office-based hysteroscopy feasible. Most importantly, hysteroscopy has significantly improved the precision of surgery by directly visualizing the surgical field. It provides superior resection of endometrial tissue and accurate lesion localization. Nowadays, hysteroscopy is used for the diagnosis and treatment of different hyperplastic and neoplastic conditions, such as the management of endometrial hyperplasia, surgical sterilization, and treatment of chronic endometritis.

7.2. Endometrial Resection or Ablation Techniques

Endometrial resection or ablation procedures can be classified as second-generation techniques. They are more conservative, largely superficial destructive interventions. Despite their effectiveness, they lack the ability to directly examine the depth of tissue destruction in real time during the procedure and are only applicable to women presenting with a normal size cavity during hysteroscopy. Since the technique bypasses the upper vagina and cervix, this hysteroscopically controlled approach can be offered in the office and in the operating room. The five variations available are performed by blowing heated humidified fluid via a hysteroscopic sheath to sear tissue and maintain cavity visualization.

This is an operative hysteroscopic approach requiring generally regional or partial anesthesia and a day or two off from work activities. The procedure combines warmth or heated fluid, preferably with simultaneous attempt at tissue desiccation or vaporization, to create some depth of endometrial destruction, resolving with direct entry into the peritoneal cavity. The technique requires assessment of the cavity, insulation of the myometrium from over-warming tissue damage, controlled depth endometrial damage, mucocoagulation avoidance, and maintenance of hysteroscopic distension. Contemporary techniques are effective with low complication rates and the ability to assess tissue for quality and adequacy of lesion formation in real time.

8. Emerging Treatment Options

Biomaterials have lately attracted much attention in relation to a woman's body. A number of promising endometrial substitutes are being developed that are behaviourally rather like the Rogers PLUS. All investigated are seen to fix well and to provide a measure of protection from the proangiogenic bioactions. Those not being re-evaluated for the BRCA1/2 carriers who seem to be dysproteinaemic are few, with even fewer, many editorialists say, that evidence-based medicine is being unreasonably sacrificed on the altar of absurd laws promulgated by 50-year-old men. There seem to be no studies even considering the benefit of genetic clotting surveillance to either the general population or to those who are actually being physically healed.

Pharmacological agents, other than for conventional contraception, are being re-evaluated for efficacy in light of the many perioperative problems first described by Rock (1978). This chapter is about manipulating the endometrium to help keep the status quo. The low price of oral contraceptives and the economic arguments for treating using devices mean that cost is unlikely to be an important factor in future decisions about the treatment or non-treatment of abnormal uterine bleeding in the early part of the second millennium after Christ. The cost-effectiveness of some of the new small molecule thrombin inhibitors, on the other hand, is still to be elucidated.

9. Management of Abnormal Uterine Bleeding in Specific Populations

The highest priority for adolescents is determining if the bleeding issue is due to abnormal endometrium tissue, which is most commonly initiated by anovulation. Once uterine pathology is ruled out, secondary investigations can be introduced. Often, a detailed history and physical examination are all that is needed to determine an appropriate path for interrogation. Family history of bleeding disorders helps clarify the diagnostic pathway. The most diagnostic labs are serum luteinizing hormone (LH), follicular stimulating hormone (FSH), thyroid-stimulating hormone (TSH), and prolactin. Ultrasound and occasionally magnetic resonance imaging (MRI) are utilized. Depending on the patient's comfort level, a sonohysterography may help show if any endometrial cavity abnormality is present. The current practice is to utilize combined oral contraceptives in heavy bleeding patients to regulate the cycles, decrease the bleeding, and minimize anovulatory cycles. There may be a role for the levonorgestrel intrauterine device in the management of heavy bleeding.

Hormonal therapy is not recommended in the treatment of von Willebrand disease (VWD) but oral desmopressin, tranexamic acid, and antifibrinolytic therapies are utilized.

Abnormal uterine bleeding (AUB) may need specific consideration depending on the age or reproductive status of the patient. There are many causes of AUB, but certain causes are more frequently found in specific populations. For example, a younger patient is more likely to have irregular ovulatory cycles, leading to uterine bleeding during the proliferative phase of the menstrual cycle. An older patient may have fibroids or endometrial hyperplasia as a cause of AUB. For many populations, cause and contributory factors can be multifactorial. For the adolescent, chronic anovulation is the most common cause of AUB. Other causes include systemic hormonal contraceptive use that suppress endometrial proliferation and thin the endometrial lining, polycystic ovary syndrome, eating disorders, hyperprolactinemia, and hypothyroidism. Uterine, ovarian, or extrauterine adenomyosis can also cause AUB. Use of trigger events through various medications in the reproductive cycle can also lead to isolated episodes of AUB in the adolescent.

9.1. Adolescents

Treatment can be conservatively managed. After ruling out pregnancy and significant medical problems (such as clotting disorders), hormone therapy should be considered if the blood loss is significant. Three proprietary progestational agents have FDA-approved labeling. All progestational agents are equally effective in stopping acute bleeding. They have equivalent action because of the common pathway of progestational medicine hormone action. However, the response is patient-dependent: there is variability among individuals, and effects are not predictable. Despite the claim of long-acting progestational agents (e.g., depomedroxyprogesterone), a patient is not reliably protected throughout the cycle from hormonal effects unless a progestational agent is given around the clock. A subsequent dose is recommended every four weeks. It is not the best approach in many cases, so compliance is often less than ideal. Comments about individual products are found in the tables in the section on medication prep.

There are no changes to the text of this section in the 2008 document.

9.2. Perimenopausal and Postmenopausal Women

It is important to rule out an endometrial carcinoma, because additional investigations such as formal dilatation and curettage or even a diagnostic hysteroscopy under general or spinal anesthesia may be performed in women with a thickened endometrium, not only in asymptomatic postmenopausal women. Lodged pieces of endometrial tissue ablation devices can migrate into the myometrium, serosal layer, broad ligament, adnexa, or even the peritoneum, causing many different out-of-pocket complications in the perimenopausal and postmenopausal women. The copper intrauterine device can effectively and safely treat heavy bleeding in perimenopausal women, as well. If conservative treatments such as progestogens or LNG-IUS fail, a careful endometrial evaluation is needed, followed by hysteroscopic removal of an intrauterine lesion with a synchronous endometrial curettage or a hysteroscopic resection for atypical hyperplasia or an endometrial carcinoma.

Perimenopausal and postmenopausal abnormal uterine bleeding is most often caused by endometrial atrophy. Dynamic contrast-enhanced magnetic resonance imaging can accurately differentiate endometrial carcinoma from endometrial atrophy in postmenopausal women with abnormal uterine bleeding, but an in-office endometrial tissue sampling, such as a Pipelle or a Karman curette, followed by endometrial histology can reliably exclude an endometrial carcinoma. Possible treatments are low-dose combined oral contraceptive pills or a cyclic hormone therapy with 200 – 400 mg vaginal micronized progesterone for 10 or 12 consecutive days, systemic hormone therapy for 10 or 14 consecutive days in each 28-day cycle, or 10 days of a combined sequential estrogen-progesterone therapy, vaginal or transdermal estrogen combined with a progestogen, and a cyclical estrogen plus intermittent progestogen therapy for 25 days each month. It is usually oral micronized progesterone, 200 mg per day for 12 consecutive days, medroxyprogesterone acetate, 10 mg per day for 10 – 14 consecutive days, or 10 mg dydrogesterone for 10 consecutive days. An intrauterine progestin-releasing system can be effective, as well.

10. Follow-Up and Monitoring of Treatment Outcomes

In general, remarking of type of lesion is proposed after treatment of adenomyosis, but on the basis that treatment is given symptomatically, rather than anatomically. Data on fibrinogen γ-chain derivatives (FGD) and immunosuppressive acidic protein (IAP) as therapy-optimizing outcome measures have been published. Three months after HIFU treatment, changes in diameter and volume (%), FGD and IAP levels (%), clotting times and pain score were significantly reduced. HIFU to treat adenomyosis is associated with a reduction in fibroid and lesion diameter and volume, with an associated fall in plasma FGD and IAP levels. These biomarker levels are acceptable therapy-optimizing outcome measures for determining adenomyosis treatment efficacy. Moreover, measurement of the plasma levels of these molecules adds an additional means of determining HIFU success.

Objective follow-up methods and standard criteria to determine treatment outcome are urgently needed. Without them, treatment for AUB is often substandard. Selection of outcome measures should both be meaningful to women and capable of revealing treatment effects. In particular, because long-term medical treatment is now a possibility, there is an urgent need for patient-centered and reliable long-term outcome measures. Relevant outcome measures for medical treatments should include satisfaction with treatment and greater treatment retention. The shortcomings of recording antibiotic prescriptions, reattendance rates, and hormones as outcome measures for long-term treatment of gynecological disease are well recognized today. An increasing amount of data indicate that satisfaction with care is closely linked with overall HRQL.

11. Complications and Adverse Effects of Treatment

Postoperative complications associated with endometrial ablation techniques can be major and may require additional surgery. Any treatment-related condition, such as endometritis, or an adverse event that prolongs the patient's recuperation, is important when the purpose of the treatment is to reduce the patient's recovery time. Such conditions may result in additional days of lost work, which might be problematic for a woman who works at a job with no leave time or because additional assistance is required for child or elder care. Other adjuvant therapy may become necessary, for example hormone replacement therapy or insertion of a copper IUD to prevent the potential for hormonal side effects.

The adverse effects associated with treatment of AUB, using medication or surgery, can be classified as minor, major, or treatment-related. One should always weigh the potential benefit of the treatment against the potential or real adverse effects. This important consideration about patient selection should be based on the likelihood of the effects as well as their potential for morbidity.

12. Patient Counseling and Education

Women with AUB should be screened for pregnancy or coexisting medical conditions. Women who have symptoms of anemia and experience heavy menstrual bleeding warrant prompt evaluation. Counseling is important as patients with AUB require time and attention to explain the laboratory, imaging, and biopsy options, as well as the treatment options. Furthermore, a patient's preferences for management should be assessed as management may be influenced by cultural or personal beliefs, and what one can tolerate and afford. Furthermore, clinicians should emphasize that new therapies that do not result in a nonfunctional endometrium do not carry the risk of endometrial cancer like hormonal therapies that result in ovulation suppression.

13. Conclusion and Future Directions

The long-term outcomes and overall effects on quality of life are, at present, uncertain. The benefits of treatment must not merely be reported but be balanced against the risks of adverse effects, particularly the effect that medical therapies have on the cause of heavy menstrual bleeding. The collective evidence that currently underpins the available treatment options often represents those of suboptimal quality. Moving forward, this evidence deficit can be corrected by providing standardization of patient symptoms and therapies with a standardized treatment regime. This collective data will then allow us to present each of the treatment options to women in the best possible way by anticipating the short-term and long-term consequences.

Although medical treatment, endometrial ablation, hysterectomy, as well as myomectomy, have all been proven effective in treating heavy menstrual bleeding, there is currently no treatment modality that is superior to the others in terms of either efficacy or patient preferences. Most of the studies had short-term follow-ups and are compromised by small patient samples, single-center nature, and selection of study population. Only long-term follow-up studies with large patient samples will effectively address these issues.

Comprehensive Guide to Treatment Options for Abnormal Uterine Bleeding

1. Introduction to Abnormal Uterine Bleeding

Abnormal uterine bleeding is excessive in duration, frequency, and quantity. It is frequent in puberty, the sexually active phase, and in the post-menopause. It has significant repercussions on quality of life, including socioprofessional issues, affecting a significant number of patients and costing several million to the healthcare system, as well as reducing the fertility indices of affected women. The definition refers mainly to the structural disorder causing the symptoms.

Abnormal uterine bleeding (AUB) in women is a common complaint in gynecology offices and emergency departments. Excessive menstrual bleeding leads to sensations of fatigue, loss of work days, limitations of daily activities, social withdrawal, and difficult domestic and professional relationships. In the past, the type of management depended on the age of the patient and on the desire for future fertility, with radical surgical treatment and hysterectomy in symptomatic women not wishing to become pregnant. Today, the objective of investigation and individualization of treatment, aiming at the improvement of the symptoms and prophylactic control of fertility, is based on the determination of circulating hormone concentrations and the prevalence of endocrine and structural disorders, and the establishment of techniques that do not interfere with the filiation function of the organ.

1.1. Definition and Prevalence

AUB presents with various symptoms and clinical signs such as the need for more or a higher absorbency of tampons and pads, regular passage of large clots in menstrual blood, or the need to double up sanitary protection. There is a profound lack of knowledge in this field among both women and health care providers. Health care practices may also lead to under-diagnosis of AUB. Only 35% of women diagnosed with AUB had sought medical care. The aim of the current review was also to enhance clinical approach to AUB by providing an understanding of how to elicit a good history, perform an appropriate physical examination, interpret laboratory and imaging findings, and institute rational patterns of treatment.

Abnormal uterine bleeding (AUB) is a frequently reported complaint and is the most common gynecological problem among women of reproductive age. The definition of AUB is based on variations in menstrual flow occurring at regular intervals. Menorrhagia, defined as excessive menstrual bleeding occurring at regular intervals, is frequently the patient's symptom. However, the duration of "normal" menstrual flow differs between ethnic groups. Up to 14 days of menstrual flow may be normal among Spanish women. The proportion of women experiencing heavy periods increases as they get older in most studies.

1.2. Classification of Abnormal Uterine Bleeding

The P component denotes structural disorders and defects: polyps (endometrial for the most part), adenomyosis, leiomyoma, and malignancy and hyperplasia. The A component denotes AUB associated with conditions or congenital uterine abnormalities, which are typically associated with hematologic dysfunction, tumor (including trophoblastic diseases), systemic disease, iatrogenic causes, coagulopathy, and ovulatory staleness or endometrial pathology. The L component denotes AUB associated with hormonal dysregulation; M denotes a key cause of AUB: whether it is related to the uterus in the form of adenomyosis or myometrial, whether it is found outside the uterus, the results are like uterine injury-related bleeding, urethral or urethral-related bleeding.

The International Federation of Gynecology and Obstetrics (FIGO) has created a system called PALM-COEIN that classifies the causes of AUB. The classification distinguishes between structural (PALM) and non-structural (COEI) causes; although these classifications are used primarily for heavy menstrual bleeding, it can also be applied to other AUB types.

2. Importance of Non-Surgical Treatment Options

There are several concepts in treating women with AUB. The first is that the condition is symptomatic and will naturally relapse after its own treatment cessation unless outflow compromise persists after treatment that requires surgery to definitively intervene. Second, medical therapy is primarily either temporary control of severe menorrhagia associated with the ovulatory cycle with the intent of prophylactic control for a defined period, or oral contraceptives may be considered. Third is that the most common cause of AUB is unknown and can become worse or spontaneously improve. When the condition does not act discreetly or solely via initiating variables supervising hemostasis in cycle control from month to month, the physician may consider a more invasive approach. Finally, consideration about the impact of different treatments on significant costs of daily living should be considered.

Abnormal uterine bleeding (AUB) is one of the most prevalent gynecologic complaints. It is the primary reason for hysterectomy in the United States and a major investigator of anemia. With safer and less invasive methods available, some non-surgical treatment options should be considered. Hysterectomy is not always necessary.

2.1. Advantages of Medication Over Surgery

In women with heavy acute bleeding, the main medical approaches are to stop the bleeding and maintain blood volume. Medical treatments are most effective if they are used as soon as the heavy bleeding starts. The most popular medications used to treat heavy bleeding are nonsteroidal anti-inflammatory drugs (NSAIDs), antifibrinolytic agents, oral progestins, and combined oral contraceptive pills. These medications are generally not associated with long-term treatment effects. The medical treatments for chronic heavy bleeding, in contrast, tend to address underlying etiologies. In women with prolonged abnormal bleeding, the focus is on conservative management. Effects on uterine bleeding are valuable, but short-term hypomenorrhea or amenorrhea does not constitute a cure. Family physicians will generally be involved in managing the effects of long-term therapy and follow up, rather than in making the definitive diagnosis and treatment choice.

Before the availability of medical therapy, uterine bleeding problems were most frequently treated with hysterectomy. Medical interventions have greatly altered the approach to abnormal uterine bleeding (AUB). The management of AUB is now focused mainly on medical intervention rather than surgical. In most women, clinical management generally does not focus on the definitive diagnosis of an underlying cause because in an office setting it is often not possible. As a result, family physicians need to understand the role of medical interventions in the assessment and management of AUB. The treatment paradigms for acute heavy bleeding and chronic AUB are different. In women with acute heavy bleeding, the medical treatment focus is on stopping the bleeding, whereas in women with chronic AUB, obtaining a gynecologic history and ordering limited diagnostic tests to rule out serious pathology is the mainstay of acute treatment prior to subsequent diagnostic testing.

3. Medication Options for Abnormal Uterine Bleeding

Therapeutic interventions address the dysfunction created by unopposed estrogen and restore hormonal control by alleviating the symptom of the erratic, uncontrolled uterine bleeding. Medical therapies can be divided into four general categories: First-line medical therapy, Second-line medical therapy, Investigational medical therapies, and Contraceptive methods and sterilization. Before initiating medications, the clinician should make sure the patient understands the potential risks and benefits of using medications and make sure the patient has been thoroughly evaluated, has an accurate diagnosis, and is an appropriate candidate for medication management.

The medical therapies for the treatment of AUB are numerous and can be as simple as over-the-counter (OTC) nonsteroidal anti-inflammatory drugs (NSAIDs) or as complex as gonadotropin-releasing hormone (GnRH) agonists, with many other options in between. Thus, we are fortunate to have a flexible medical armamentarium of AUB treatments. The medical armamentarium for treating AUB is wide and deserves careful consideration.

3.1. Nonsteroidal Anti-Inflammatory Drugs (NSAIDs)

Misoprostol is an orally active prostaglandin E2 analogue. Studies have shown that it reduces blood loss dramatically. It has been observed that it has an excellent effect on the prevention of ovulation. It is an effective second-line drug for immediate control of severe symptoms. Although misoprostol is an effective treatment, there is not enough evidence of its effect on menstrual pain. It is used to stop bleeding and reduce bleeding in resource-wealthy areas. Its rapid effect can be felt in about 2 h. If used in doses of 200–800 µg, it can be effective. Its properties include improving contraceptive efficacy with minimal impairment of reproduction and easy shopping and storage. Its use is limited in women who have not given birth and have not experienced a uterine abortion because it has been shown to increase the prevalence of uterine contractions. Its contractions result in a prolonged process and, after delivery, it results in less increase in the hemoglobin of the body of the patient. Its unwanted effects can give menstrual pain, nausea, vomiting, diarrhea, fever, headache, and sleepiness. Women are required to use barrier contraception or are supplied with their desire to have offspring or sterilize.

The most effective first-line prophylactic treatment is a high dose of NSAIDs used for at least 5–6 days, given every 6–8 h. It is at least as effective as hormone therapy. Research has shown that NSAID dosing convenience and efficacy have better therapeutic results. For some patients, adverse effects such as gastric complaints, heartburn, upset stomach, an unwanted increase in blood pressure, headaches, and hypersensitivity are seen. The American College of Obstetricians and Gynecologists recommended the use of NSAIDs only if a side effect of menses leads to functional impairment. The use of intermittent NSAIDs for 2–3 days for patients who are satisfied with this treatment is found to be adequate and tolerable. Minimal use of this drug is more precious. NSAID use may also be beneficial due to the anti-inflammatory effect in cases where the pain becomes excessive.

Nonsteroidal anti-inflammatory drugs (NSAIDs) such as mefenamic acid, ibuprofen, and naproxen have been used to control somatic pain for a long time. Their role in controlling bleeding is related to their effect on prostaglandins. NSAIDs inhibit the production of prostaglandins by blocking the cyclooxygenase enzyme that is important for the production of prostaglandins beneath the endometrium. If prostaglandins are not produced by endometrial cells, local vasoconstriction occurs. The prostanoid enhances the contracting effect of ergotonine and enhances the anti-aggregant effect of antidiuretic hormones which give bleeding control. NSAIDs reduce the blood loss by half but they have to be used for 6 days at regular intervals and produce many cyclooxygenase enzyme synthesis effects depending on doses.

3.2. Hormonal Therapies

As in many gynecologic diagnoses, treatment of AUB begins with a hormonal approach. While hormonal treatment is not definitive therapy such as surgery, D&C, or hysteroscopy, it usually is pursued for several months before further treatment. In many cases, menstrual bleeding can become normal after cessation of hormone therapy; the bleeding caused by anovulation may only require time to self-correct. For DUB, additional therapy is traditionally reserved for only those who are symptomatic and require treatment. However, even in the presence of structural lesions such as polyps, fibroids, or adenomyosis, hormonal therapy may be able to control symptoms and prevent surgery if the patient has not already completed her family.

This is a broad, comprehensive review of current therapies for abnormal uterine bleeding. This review encompasses medical, surgical, and interventional treatment options. This is based on published literature and expert opinion, where evidence-based data is limited. We have started with a discussion on flexible endometrial ablation—most promising at this time, and moving to non-hysteroscopic ablation techniques, hysteroscopic resection of endometrium and fibroids, ablation and resection of adenomyosis, and non-endometrial sources of uterine bleeding. We felt that it was essential to discuss these feasible options and complications thoroughly.

4. Non-Medication Treatment Options

Uterine fibroid HIFU offers patients with a layer of intervention without risk of complications or pain that is enough to be lived through without the healthcare practitioner. During HIFU solutions, high-grade ultrasound energy is transported through the passages to the required site and allows beams of cold flesh melt the tissue of the fibroid nuclei. With ultrasonic imaging, physicians can monitor the transformation. At a localized level, uterine fibroids are destroyed. Prospective studies demonstrated that symptom development and quality of life stayed stable in 89% of individuals at 2 years after treatment. Their study showed, however, that ultrasounded AUB pre-operative results can make it very hard to safely handle HIFU on its own.

High-Intensity Focused Ultrasound

The success of uterine artery embolization in improving bleeding adhered to reducing bulk symptoms resulting from symmetrical myomas. Please see the detailed study about Uterine Artery Embolization post.

Uterine Artery Embolization

Myomectomy remains the cornerstone of surgical management of symptomatic fibroids in patients desiring fertility. This is an extremely intricate, painful, and significant operation with risks and implications. Uterine adenoid tumors have primarily been done with open surgical methods historically.

Myomectomy

Dilation and curettage has long been a traditional form of therapy for the management of AUB, and with some practitioners still using it about 15% of the time, based on a prospective survey at a large academic institution. The relaxation of the cervix is associated with the induction of general anesthesia or IV sedation, which is associated with significant morbidity. Therefore, other treatments that do not require hospital operating.

Dilation and Curettage

Since a number of medical therapy options are available for the management of abnormal uterine bleeding, we will focus here on non-medication options for therapy.

Introduction

4.1. Endometrial Ablation

Endometrial ablation technologies are relatively new. These methods are being used more frequently as an alternative to hysterectomy. Before the menstrual disorders that women experiencing abnormal bleeding have are treated with one of these technologies, medications can be used for both diagnostic and therapeutic purposes. These endometrial ablation techniques ablate and destroy thin layers of the endometrium in a variety of ways. Some techniques use the application of hot or cold technologies, i.e. laser, microwave, radio frequency electrical energy, or cryoablation. In a few techniques, the endometrium is vaporized. There is one technique that separates and crushes the endometrial components – the Novasure treatment.

Endometrial ablation, the physical ablation and/or destruction of the uterine lining, has three advantages over other treatment options for abnormal uterine bleeding. First, women are usually treated in an outpatient office setting as opposed to an ambulatory surgical setting. Second, this treatment does not destroy the uterus itself, and the procedure potentially allows a woman to maintain her fertility. Third, the risk of complication from this procedure is also lower than seen in hysterectomy. Matic et al. estimate a 0.8% DVT rate, a 1.5% risk of hemorrhage, and a 1.5% infection risk when three of these procedures are performed. The complication rate from endometrial ablation cannot be expressed as a percentage for it varies based on the various endometrial ablation technologies used.

4.2. Uterine Artery Embolization

There are also some complications from UAE, including but not limited to nontarget embolization, infection, and necrosis of the lower urinary tract, or delayed retroperitoneal hematoma. In a systematic review of 381 women who had UAE for symptomatic fibroids and presented data regarding urinary symptomatology before and after embolization, such as urinary retention, dysuria, urinary frequency, or urinary incontinence, it was found that the mean improvement for the seven studies was 67%. The factors that increase postembolization syndrome include having a submucosal fibroid, volume of devascularized fibroids, and method of UAE. Patients also expressed a preference for uterus preservation in fertility desire.

Uterine artery embolization (UAE) is a minimally invasive therapy that has been widely performed for the treatment of uterine fibroids since the late 1990s. Current indications for UAE have been expanded to not only uterine fibroids but also to abnormal uterine bleeding (AUB), uterine adenomyosis, and placenta accreta. UAE is a radiologically guided procedure that leads to a transient ischemic necrosis of the uterine myomas. There are a myriad of reported studies underlining the efficacy and safety of UAE. The efficacy rate of UAE to control menorrhagia or hypermenorrhea caused by fibroids is 80-95%, and the technical success rate of UAE is high (95-99%). The overall major complication rate is reported to be less than 2.4% in some systematic reviews. The most common symptom after UAE related to the patient's quality of life is postembolization syndrome, which includes moderate to severe pain requiring opiates, fever, and postembolization symptoms including pain and fever together. The readmission rate is 8-10%.

5. Combination Therapies

5.2. Combined Hormonal Treatment Although it can be difficult for a patient to endure side effects, along with the estrogenic action, the serum levels of estrogen when combined with a progestin, acting synergistically, makes toleration easier for the patient. Additionally, the preoperative estrogen therapy induces a three-to-fourfold increase in vascularity and alters the tissue component of fibroids, which ultimately result in easier vaginal procedures, lower complication rates, decreased uterine infection rate, and decreased blood loss. These effects are less pronounced for the DRSP than for NETA or LET, whereas anti-inflammatory effects are stronger in terms of its effect, and its nausea status is relatively less than the other combined forms. Devices acting as systems, including the progestin-eluting IUD and progestin injections, in combination with the NETA pill, resulted in a gain of improvement in bleeding duration, especially for women over 35 years of age with improvement in the duration of bleeding over 25 days, the follicular phase days.

5.1. Combined Antifibrinolytics and Progestin

The combination of antifibrinolytics and progestin is an extremely safe combination of both medications. Besides bleeding reduction, it has an anti-inflammatory effect, which is important not only for reducing the production of pain during the bleeding but causing a direct action and reducing the pelvic pain status related to its anti-inflammatory effect. With hormonal therapy, there are other menstrual cycle-related symptoms such as breast tenderness, which are typical but bearable symptoms for the patients taking a progestin for mild AUB as well as women looking for a pill or other hormonal method of contraception.

Although combination therapy has not really lived up to its potential, in many cases - cyclical hormonal therapy combined with other therapies, the combination of a mechanical device with a hormone medication - shows great promise for the future. The DRSP in oral contraceptives combined with Ulipristal showed results on quality of life and symptom control for bleeding. Levonorgestrel intrauterine system and a GnRH agonist make the 12 weeks pretreatment feasible, fully enhance the progestogen effect, and maintain the remission from heavy menstrual bleeding by continuing the LNG-IUS after the completion of GnRH agonist therapy. Thus, combination therapies of different therapies resulting in the global improvement on the symptomatology of AUB in a harm-free situation deserve a more comprehensive study.

5.1. Benefits and Considerations

Abnormal uterine bleeding (AUB) is a high-risk medical condition that requires prompt, accurate, and compassionate management of the patient. Physical findings are often benign, but to diagnose and treat the underlying etiology, various gynecologic tests (such as laboratory tests, ultrasound, hysteroscopy, and endometrial biopsy) may be uncomfortable, and physical findings may be embarrassing. The gynecologist should be alert to the patient's needs and respectful of their personal dignity. Treatment options include patient-based pharmacologic therapy and operative interventions (both inpatient and outpatient). The increasing availability of medication, especially oral contraceptive pills, makes it possible for many women to manage their disease without hormonal therapy, thus, underscoring an in-depth investigation of the agents used in this review as well as investigational agents that are in development. The methods of treatment are constantly being refined, and they will continue to suggest women a wider variety of safe and effective options for the management of AUB.

Oral contraceptives are widely accepted as first-line therapy for women with symptoms of excessive uterine bleeding who want to avoid pregnancy. The benefits include a regular source of medication, reduced menstrual bleeding, improved dysmenorrhea, and the added benefit of contraception. Some studies have shown an increased risk of anemia in women with prolonged or heavy menstrual flow compared with women without increased bleeding, which suggests a potential protective effect of COC (combined oral contraceptive) method use against high levels of menstrual bleeding. In addition, some estrogen-progestin regimens are FDA-approved for treating DUB. However, some women have underlying conditions that preclude taking the estrogen component of COCs, which is progesterone therapy undertaken in such women. The woman must also accept potential irregular bleeding associated with the use of these agents and undergo regular pregnancy evaluations.

For all of the hormonal interventions, decision points include the woman's desire for regular menstrual bleeding; if the condition is accompanied by symptoms related to the menstrual cycle, the individual woman's ability to tolerate and adhere to medication taken for a cycle-related condition, and the need for alternate contraception.

6. Patient Counseling and Shared Decision-Making

Short-term management interventions can stop bleeding and can be an important provider strategy for engaging in shared decision-making with the patient. Such a pause in bleeding will offer patients the opportunity to consult with their healthcare provider during a bleeding cessation. With the creation of this document, providers can maintain the discussion and shared decision-making process prior to long-term comprehensive management. When treatment is successful, patients will benefit and the healthcare system will save costs. It is important to consider aspects of access to care, treatment acceptability, treatment burden, contraceptive benefit, systemic effects, and the necessity for future fertility in selecting a treatment plan. A variety of treatment options provide acceptable bleeding outcomes.

When treating patients with abnormal uterine bleeding, it is important to meet patient preferences and treatment expectations. Patients should be educated regarding the risks, benefits, side effects, and costs of treatment to support the shared decision-making process. More satisfactory clinical management is often provided to patients participating in shared decision-making. The patient should be offered various medical and surgical treatment options that match the patient's preference. A thorough patient discussion can help tailor treatment. Patients have a better understanding of the desired method of treatment and have higher satisfaction over the long term by developing a treatment plan that meets the patient's personal goals.

6.1. Importance of Informed Consent

It is supposed that a prerequisite for the choice of a treatment method for a patient with bleeding dysfunction is to determine the necessity or undesirability of preserving the possibility of subsequent childbearing. The main sampling algorithm is to determine the sanogenous state of the uterus. Determination of the sanogenous state of the uterus is limited by the few existing instrumental methods.

In view of the importance of the patient's informed consent for choosing a method of treatment, informing the patient of the features and possible complications of treatment is also the main activity of the doctor. The physician is not supposed to only give the patient all the necessary information and allow her to decide on the method for solving her problem. This is also a legal obligation of the physician. It is desirable for the patient to be advised in a sufficiently broad manner to make informed consent. The patient must thoroughly digest all the information received and provide the doctor with some additional questions. Only after that the patient will make a fully conscious and free decision. Patient informed consent for the chosen treatment method blocks the absence of the patient's negative attitude to the planned manipulations in the postoperative period.

7. Follow-Up and Monitoring

Patients who have undergone minimally invasive uterine sparing procedures such as endometrial ablation may require follow-up imaging studies of the uterus to confirm normal involution and complete resolution of the myomas located in the uterine wall. Suggested preoperative work-up or selection of patients for hysterectomy is discussed above. Appropriate counseling is also essential to set realistic expectations of the outcome of the therapy. A comprehensive consultation for the patient at the time of the initial visit and the regular follow-up visits is recommended. Information regarding potential side effects after therapy and instructions for reporting them should be addressed. Most practitioners use a standardized questionnaire for recording the information.

To achieve effective and favorable treatment results, patients must be monitored for follow-up. It is important that the patient understands the need for the follow-up visits. Some patients tend to overlook these appointments since they feel well after the initial response to treatment and the early perioperative period. Patients who are treated with oral medications may not complete the full course of therapy and may have a tendency to underreport the coexisting menstrual-related symptoms. They may require additional counseling regarding the possibility of future pregnancy and contraceptive methods if needed. They should be advised that fertility is frequently restored once the abnormal uterine bleeding has been treated, particularly when the size of the uterus is not markedly increased.

7.1. Key Parameters to Monitor

However, adenomyomectomy or myomectomy is difficult after endometrial ablation, with either laser endometrial ablation at the time of myomectomy being more important, or pretreatment with GnRH agonist to decrease myoma size, will be required in the future desired fertility. Subsequent pain may be due to post-endometrial ablation tubal sterility with possible tubal distention or cornual agglutination. These different types of postablation tubal sterilization and subsequent treatment are important to acknowledge because the etiology will affect future desired fertility and later treatments. Patients who undergo any ablation technique should be counseled and monitored about risk factors for, and symptoms of thermal injury before and after global endometrial ablation or thermal endometrial ablation.

Post-endometrial ablation procedures, long-term annual follow-ups can be beneficial as they have shown that 21% to 27% of women required re-treatment or hysterectomy over 4-7 years. The most common reasons for hysterectomy following rollerball ablation are pelvic pain, subsequent bleeding, endometrial regrowth or hysterectomy for small fibroids which were previously asymptomatic and found incidentally at the time of follow-up. Some patients with previous rollerball ablation cause difficulty with subsequent surgery due to the small holes from previous rollerball ablation. If pregnancy is the patient's desire, this may be a significant potential risk. The most common indication in women with previous global endometrial ablation is pelvic pain (including pelvic cramping or severe menstrual-like pain or cramping) due to adenomyosis-specific pain or dysfunction.